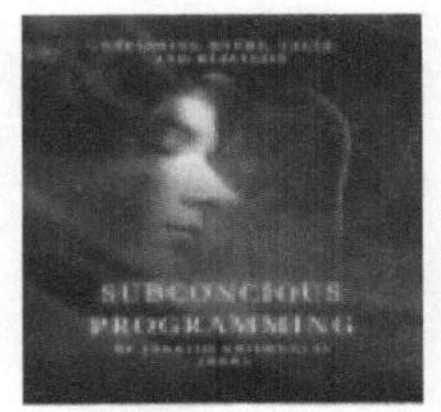
SUBCONCIOUS
PROGRAMMING

I0844733

While every precaution has been taken in the preparation of this book, the publisher assumes no responsibility for errors or omissions, or for damages resulting from the use of the information contained herein.

SUBCONCIOUS PROGRAMMING

First edition. January 6, 2024.

Written by Jagdish Krishanlal Arora.

Also by Jagdish Krishanlal Arora

Basic Inorganic and Organic Chemistry
Book of Jokes
Car Insurance and Claims
Digital Electronics, Computer Architecture and
Microprocessor Design Principles
Guided Meditation and Yoga
The Bible and Jesus Christ
Unity Quest
From Oasis to Global Stage: The Evolution of Arab
Civilization
Secrets of Mount Kailash, Bermuda Triangle and the
Lost City of Atlantis
Visitors from Outer Space
Motivation
The Aliens and God Theory
The Lunar Voyager
Queen Elizabeth II and the British Monarchy
The Kremlin Conspiracy
Vegetable Gardening, Salads and Recipes
How to End The War in Ukraine
The Old and New World Order
Travelling to Mars in the Cosmic Odyssey 2050
Romance Pays Off
How the Universe Works
Mental Health and Well Being
Ancient History of Mars
The Nexus
Basic and Advanced Physics
Administrative Law

Calculus
The Ramayana
A Watery Mystery
Romantic Conflicts
Thieves of Palestine
Love in Chicago
WordPress Design and Development
Travellers Guide to Mount Kailash
Become a Better Writer With Creative Writing
Emerging Trends in Carbon Emission Reduction
India Independence Through Non Violence
Copyright, Patents, Trademarks and Trade Secret Laws
Decoding CHATGPT and Artificial Intelligence
The Untold Story of Diana and Prince Charles
Time Travel
How to Lose Weight Quickly
Subconcious Programming

Table of Contents

SUBCONCIOUS PROGRAMMING

Exploring Myths, Facts and Realties

BY

JAGDISH KRISHANLAL ARORA

techbagg@outlook.com

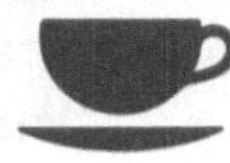

Introduction

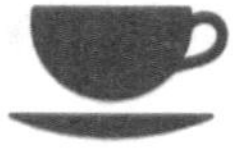

THE PEOPLE WHO TEACH subconscious programming themselves have never achieved it themselves. The reason is that not everyone can achieve sub-conscious programming. In one project they were offering one million dollars to give code for how cells operate. The reason for me not giving that kind of information is that is it too dangerous to give that kind of knowledge, secondly it was a open source competition and thirdly on one NASA project where I gave design for a vacuum garbage collector and ejector I did not get the price of 10,000 dollars as they said I need to make an American a partner in the project in one week so I did not get the money.

Only partial control of the sub-conscious is possible and the sub-conscious is hugely resistant to change and stubborn. We cannot change it forcefully as it is carried over from our parents who carried it from their parents and it is very old since the time humans were born. It will never allow us to see into it and what it has stored in the last 10,000 years in it.

The sub-conscious mind passes on from generation to generation and gets passed on to our siblings. A sibling may be less intelligent than us but it does not mean his sub-conscious is weak. That is the reason our views are never the same. If we did not carry information from our parents, we would just become robots and have the same views and speak the same things over and over again. Our sub-conscious mind helps us to act different from others.

Over a period of time some information in our brain changes depending on our experiences that leads to pollution which then makes brothers and sisters having different views from each other over a period of several years.

As science develops and artificial intelligence takes over, our sub-conscious power will reduce. We will be more dependent on artificial intelligence resulting in our own mind taking the back seat and becoming less productive.

The sub-conscious is most active when we are asleep and dreams serve as the backbone of sub-conscious to communicate with our conscious mind. Not all warnings in the dreams are true and we have to use our judgements to analyse the warnings in the dreams.

The sub-conscious does not communicate with us directly and it transfers information through dreams creating visual representation and stories. During the sleep process when we are dreaming the sub-conscious is also repairing and fixing our body and the dreams does not mean all that was shown was true but it was a way to give us rest while the body was repairing itself and cooling off from the day's tiredness.

I only wish that someday my powers come back and I can transfer all of the information to everyone about the human body and everything around us. Writing everything is a very tedious task.

The concept of the subconscious mind has evolved significantly over time, from ancient philosophical musings to the groundbreaking theories of Freud, Jung, and other influential thinkers. Their contributions shaped the foundation of modern psychology, paving the way for continued exploration and understanding of the intricate workings of the human mind.

The conscious and subconscious minds operate in a complex and intertwined manner, jointly shaping human behaviour, perceptions, and decision-making processes. Acknowledging their distinct functions and understanding how they interact empowers individuals to navigate their thoughts and actions more effectively, fostering personal growth and self-improvement.

First, we will understand what is in our mind and its parts. After we have fully understood how our brain is made and its structure, we will go onto the depts of sub-conscious programming.

Our sub-conscious or consciousnesses are also connected to the entire world and maybe we communicate with each other when we breathe in and out the common air around us. Our thoughts change dramatically as we move away from our village, town and city and they do not remain the same after we leave those places for a very long time.

The sub-conscious mind can solve critical diseases and has a large capacity to solve various mysteries. Through its will power it can cure illness that are not possible by modern medicines but it also requires the intake of necessary proteins, vitamins and other healthy foods.

The sub-conscious will not work to cure a disease or be programmed without a proper nutritious diet.

Meditation and yoga are just partial reliefs and it no way affect the sub-consciousness. If they were real the sadhus and rishis who practised them 2000 years back would have been great people. The tradition of yoga and meditation continues to this day but you will see most of the people who do them are unclad or half-clad people in India surviving by begging on the roads for alms.

Those who claim our mind becomes superior by yoga and meditation are themselves becoming weak and desperate themselves. Yoga and meditation are only an avenue for getting relief from stress and not something that will make us more intelligent or strong in the body. They are just like any cardio, aerobic, and PT exercises.

We have so many books of ancient times like Ramayana and Mahabharata which speak of which claim of use of powerful weapons and aircrafts existing 2000 years back, also in Egyptian and Greek mythology but there are no records and traces of them anywhere on stones, statues or in cave drawings.

The UFOs we see today are the same people claimed to have seen 2000-5000 years back which means the aliens never advanced in technology and the humans have developed technology faster than aliens. Does sub-consciousness have a role in this or is it evolution or some big bang theory taking place developing science and modern medicine.

We have still not evolved from man being created or evolving from monkeys, and big bang theory creating the universe and life generating from bacteria over trillions of years. Nobody asked how did bacteria come or something became bacteria. The same question did the chicken come first or the eggs.

The angels and guides we speak of is nothing but the sub-conscious mind. If it is highly developed it will guide us properly and if its stored experiences are bad, it will misguide us.

The spinal cord has nothing to do with kundalini it is all fake and the spinal cord transmits signals from the brain as well as it transfers energy and electrical signals. The kundalini mentioned in some religious texts does not exist but because the humans of those times were unaware of the sub-consciousness mind operating through the pineal and pituitary gland.

There is no such thing such as third eye and it is only the functioning of the sub-consciousness and the pineal and pituitary gland.

The pineal gland, often referred to as the pineal body or epiphysis cerebri, is a tiny, cone-shaped structure situated at the posterior region of the brain's third ventricle. Comprised of portions of neurons, neuroglial cells, and specialized secretory cells known as pinacocytes, this gland is responsible for the production and secretion of melatonin, a hormone that regulates the sleep-wake cycle and plays a role in various physiological functions, including circadian rhythms and reproductive hormone modulation. Despite its small size, the pineal gland plays a crucial role in regulating certain bodily processes and maintaining biological rhythms.

While both the pituitary gland and the pineal gland are crucial components of the endocrine system, their roles and functions differ. The pituitary gland, often referred to as the "master gland," is responsible for producing and releasing a wide array of hormones that regulate various bodily functions, including growth, reproduction, metabolism, and stress response. It consists of two main parts: the anterior pituitary (adenohypophysis) and the posterior pituitary (neurohypophysis). The anterior pituitary synthesizes and releases hormones like growth hormone, prolactin, thyroid-stimulating hormone, adrenocorticotropic hormone, follicle-stimulating hormone, and luteinizing hormone, among others, affecting functions such as growth, lactation, metabolism, and reproduction. The posterior pituitary, on the other hand, stores and releases hormones produced in the hypothalamus, such as oxytocin and vasopressin, which regulate behaviours related to bonding, love, and stress responses.

On the other hand, the pineal gland is responsible for the secretion of melatonin, primarily involved in regulating the sleep-wake cycle (circadian rhythms). Melatonin production by the pineal gland is affected by the exposure to light and darkness and plays a crucial role in maintaining the body's internal clock, influencing sleep patterns and other biological rhythms.

While the pituitary gland plays a role in the release of hormones related to stress, love, and bonding (through hormones like oxytocin), the pineal gland's primary function revolves around melatonin production and the regulation of circadian rhythms. Both glands are integral parts of the endocrine system, but they have distinct roles in hormone regulation and bodily functions.

It will take a very long time to remove all superstitious build through thousands of books and videos about the third eye, meditation, yoga and other fictions. If it were true, the people of those religions would have created UFOs, flying aircrafts and superior weapons much before we created them now.

Some of the concepts are true but are available only to selective human beings but it is not an inherent part of every human body but an extra feature in special type of human beings. It cannot be added or modified using subconscious programming. That is why even after thousands of years of meditation and yoga the sadhus and rishis of today are not having those powers or knowledge.

For example, I have those features but they are not active in me or they will remain inactive till such time I am on this planet. I wrote about artificial intelligence in 2015 but it has become a reality today and when it was told in the 1960s no one knew what it meant that time I was not born.

I was very knowledgeable in all these spiritual things at 10 years of age, but it took me a long time to get good grades in school and college in school and college subjects. Even after I knew everything about the universe and body, mind and spirit it did not help me get good grades till final years of my college when I got 88 % in final semester.

But my mind guided me over the years to learn everything that Earth has stored over the last 10,000 years, all of the history, civilizations, technologies, everything possible. But I am not a master in everything know only a few programming languages, technologies, and human languages. I am still not able to work like a supercomputer or open my third eye or the kundalini hoaxes even after having gained unlimited knowledge and knowing entire thing about the human body and how it functions and operates.

I don't consider my third eye and kundalini opened for several reasons. On our planet the third eye functions in a different way, it imparts us knowledge and instant answers and helps us communicate correctly through telepathy. The kundalini transmits electrical signals and information using our conscious commands on our planet. But in humans these functions occur through the sub-conscious mind and that is why I said these features have not been given to your human bodies.

At first, I was afraid of activating my powers on your planet I my human body but over the time have realised that it may not be possible to activate it on your planet even if I had tried. If my powers activate on your planet, it would be a miracle. I also believe that the human body operates by sunlight and solar energy and my concept will be accepted by humans over a period of time.

The Hindus, Buddhist sadhus and rishis and people of other religions were only trying to tap the sub-conscious mind to get something unique out of it. The aliens also believe the human sub-conscious mind is the spirit in inactive state which means even the aliens are ignorant about it and consider it to be super powerful which it is not.

The sub-conscious is not super powerful and even 500 years ahead it will remain the same. Programming it means we can only use it to gain knowledge, improve ourselves and lead a more meaningful life. I cannot make you superhumans through subconscious programming.

Neither the Vedas, or other religious texts or future technologies can make you or me super human. While on earth I analysed all of these things and found only my spiritual power from my own planet can make me super human and there is nothing on earth which can convert me to an extraordinary being. Those features if they ever existed were removed from earth and those extraordinary features were there only in our beings who either came from our planet or were born to women on this planet from marriage to people from our exoplanets as they are called on earth.

But exploring your sub-conscious mind will help you to self-realise yourself better and it is not permanent. The day you stop exploring it goes back to its inactive state.

Understanding Subconscious Programming

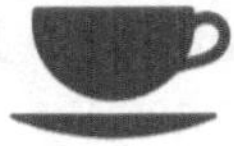

THE INFLUENCE OF SUBCONSCIOUS Programming on Human Behaviour

Subconscious programming is a powerful force that significantly impacts human behaviour and perception. It operates beneath the surface of conscious awareness, shaping our thoughts, beliefs, and actions in ways we may not readily recognize. Understanding its formation, mechanisms, and significance is crucial in comprehending how it affects our lives.

Formation of Subconscious Programs

The genesis of subconscious programming can be traced back to various factors that mould our experiences and beliefs. Childhood experiences play a pivotal role, as they lay the foundation for many subconscious patterns. The interactions, teachings, and environments during formative years contribute significantly to the creation of these subconscious programs. Moreover, societal norms, cultural influences, and social conditioning further shape our subconscious, instilling beliefs and behaviours that often operate automatically without conscious thought.

Mechanisms of Subconscious Programming

Subconscious programming employs multiple mechanisms to embed itself in our minds. Repetition is a fundamental aspect, as experiences or information encountered frequently tend to become ingrained in our subconscious. Emotional intensity also plays a crucial role; events or experiences that evoke strong emotions have a more profound impact on subconscious programming. Furthermore, sensory input, encompassing what we see, hear, feel, smell, and taste, actively influences our subconscious, creating associations and triggers that affect our responses and behaviours.

The Significance of Subconscious Programming

The significance of subconscious programming lies in its influence on our perceptions and decision-making processes. It shapes how we view the world, impacting our attitudes, beliefs, and interpretations of events. Moreover, it exerts a profound effect on decision-making, often guiding our choices without explicit conscious consideration. By acknowledging the role of subconscious programming, individuals can begin to comprehend their behavioural patterns and reactions, allowing for introspection and potential changes in behaviour.

In essence, subconscious programming is a multifaceted process with far-reaching implications for human behaviour. Acknowledging its existence and understanding its mechanisms empowers individuals to take control of their thoughts and behaviours. Through this awareness, one can consciously evaluate and modify subconscious programs, leading to positive transformations and improved decision-making.

Taking charge of subconscious programming involves practices such as mindfulness, self-reflection, and deliberate exposure to new ideas or experiences. By consciously engaging with these practices, individuals can gradually rewire their subconscious patterns, fostering personal growth and enhancing their overall well-being.

In conclusion, the influence of subconscious programming is profound, shaping our perceptions, beliefs, and behaviours in ways that often elude conscious recognition. Understanding its formation, mechanisms, and significance enables individuals to navigate their subconscious landscape effectively, fostering personal development and creating opportunities for positive change.

Techniques for Subconscious Reprogramming

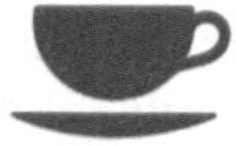

THE HUMAN MIND OPERATES on multiple levels, with subconscious programming serving as a fundamental mechanism that shapes our thoughts, beliefs, and actions without our conscious awareness. Understanding this process is essential as it significantly impacts our perception of the world and guides our decision-making.

Formation of Subconscious Programs

Subconscious programming is intricately woven from various sources, primarily stemming from our formative years. Childhood experiences hold immense influence, imprinting patterns of thought and behaviour that endure into adulthood. These early encounters, coupled with social conditioning and cultural norms, contribute to the formation of deep-seated subconscious programs. As these experiences and influences persist and accumulate, they solidify into automatic responses, shaping our perspectives and actions.

Mechanisms of Subconscious Programming

The subconscious mind functions as a repository of absorbed information, employing diverse mechanisms to process and retain data. Repetition is a key driver; information encountered repeatedly becomes ingrained, guiding our subconscious reactions. Emotional intensity serves as another potent influencer, as experiences laden with strong emotions leave lasting imprints on our subconscious. Additionally, sensory input what we see, hear, feel, taste, and smell constantly feeds our subconscious, constructing associations and triggers that influence our perceptions and behaviours.

The Significance of Subconscious Programming

The impact of subconscious programming is far-reaching, significantly moulding how we interpret the world and make decisions. It forms the lens through which we view reality, shaping our beliefs, attitudes, and responses. Often operating beneath conscious thought, these programmed patterns guide our choices and behaviours. Recognizing this influence allows individuals to gain control over their subconscious processes, enabling deliberate modifications that lead to positive changes in behaviour and outlook.

In short, subconscious programming profoundly shapes our cognition and behaviour. Acknowledging its formation from childhood experiences, social conditioning, and cultural influences illuminates the origins of our subconscious programs. Understanding the mechanisms repetition, emotional intensity, and sensory input provides insight into how these programs are established and maintained. Realizing the significance of subconscious programming empowers individuals to consciously influence their thoughts and behaviours, fostering personal growth and facilitating constructive changes in their lives.

Making the primitive humans intelligent was very difficult during the stone age. They became barbarians, hunted animals, ate each other to survive and had to be tamed. They were taught using symbols and hand gestures and even after so much advancement the humans are very much different from the aliens.

Now after so many years of writing I am able to tell how humans were made and developed which was impossible to tell only 10 years back.

T

Reprogramming the Subconscious Mind and Unveiling Limiting Beliefs

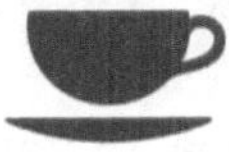

THE SUBCONSCIOUS MIND serves as an intricate framework that shapes our beliefs, behaviours, and actions. Often operating beneath conscious awareness, it harbours entrenched patterns of thought that can either propel us forward or hinder our progress. Identifying and reprogramming these subconscious elements are pivotal steps towards fostering personal growth and achieving our aspirations.

Identifying Limiting Beliefs

Limiting beliefs act as invisible barriers that obstruct our potential and impede our progress towards self-fulfilment. Originating from childhood experiences and reinforced through repeated encounters and societal influences, these beliefs significantly influence our decisions and behaviours. Recognizing them represents the initial stride towards reprogramming the subconscious mind. Diverse methods aid in unearthing and pinpointing these concealed convictions residing within the subconscious realm.

Journaling emerges as a potent tool in uncovering limiting beliefs. Writing down thoughts, emotions, and recurrent patterns illuminates underlying beliefs that might otherwise remain concealed. It provides a tangible record that aids in analysing and understanding the origins and impact of these beliefs. Additionally, meditation acts as a gateway to explore the subconscious landscape. Through introspection and focused attention, one can delve deeper into the mind, unveiling hidden beliefs and examining their roots.

Collaborating with a therapist or counsellor also proven invaluable in identifying and challenging limiting beliefs. Trained professionals guide individuals through self-exploration, offering insights and strategies to confront and reframe these ingrained convictions. By acknowledging and challenging these beliefs, individuals initiate the process of liberating themselves from their restrictive hold, thereby paving the way for embracing new patterns of thought and behaviour.

Mindfulness and Awareness Practices

Mindfulness and awareness practices serve as potent allies in the quest to reprogram the subconscious mind. Embracing mindfulness involves cultivating a heightened sense of awareness in the present moment. Techniques such as meditation, deep breathing exercises, and body scanning facilitate the observation and examination of subconscious thoughts and reactions. By fostering mindfulness, individuals disrupt established subconscious patterns, creating an opening for reprogramming.

Awareness acts as a cornerstone in the journey of subconscious reprogramming. By consciously observing thoughts and behaviours, individuals gain insights into their internal processes, enabling the identification of repetitive patterns. This heightened awareness empowers individuals to consciously choose their responses and actions, steering away from limiting beliefs and fostering new, positive thought patterns.

Affirmations, Visualization, and Repetition

Affirmations and visualization stand as powerful tools in rewiring the subconscious mind. Affirmations, positive statements reiterated to oneself, serve to reinforce new beliefs and thought patterns. These statements, when repeated consistently, establish new neural pathways in the brain, supporting positive changes. Visualization, the process of creating mental images of desired outcomes, complements affirmations by embedding these visions into the subconscious, fostering a sense of familiarity and achievability.

Repetition serves as a critical component in reprogramming the subconscious mind. Consistently reinforcing new beliefs and thought patterns through repetition ensures their integration into subconscious programming, facilitating enduring transformations in thought and behaviour. This practice fortifies the foundations of positive change, solidifying new patterns that gradually overshadow limiting beliefs.

The subconscious mind holds immense influence over our lives, directing our thoughts, decisions, and actions. Uncovering and challenging limiting beliefs represent crucial steps towards initiating change and growth. Techniques encompassing mindfulness, awareness, affirmations, visualization, and repetition serve as guiding tools in the endeavour to reprogram the subconscious mind. By incorporating these methodologies into daily life, individuals embark on a transformative journey, breaking free from limiting beliefs and forging new paths towards a more fulfilling and empowered existence.

Applying Subconscious Programming in Daily Life

1. CREATING EMPOWERING Habits
  - Discussing how habits are formed and how subconscious programming can aid in developing positive habits.
  - Providing strategies to replace negative habits with beneficial ones through subconscious reprogramming.
  2. Enhancing Performance and Self-Improvement
  - Exploring how subconscious programming can optimize performance in various areas of life, such as career, sports, or creativity.
  - Techniques for boosting self-confidence, motivation, and achieving goals through subconscious reprogramming.
  3. Maintaining Subconscious Health and Well-being
  - Addressing the role of subconscious programming in mental health and well-being.
  - Providing guidance on utilizing subconscious techniques for stress reduction, relaxation, and emotional balance.
  What is the Subconscious Mind?
  The subconscious mind represents the part of our mental functioning that operates below the level of conscious awareness. It encompasses thoughts, feelings, desires, and memories that influence our behaviour without us actively being aware of them.

This aspect of the mind stores information, processes emotions, and controls automatic bodily functions.

While the conscious mind involves thoughts and perceptions, we are aware of, the subconscious operates in the background, influencing our thoughts, actions, and behaviours without our explicit recognition. It's like the vast reservoir of information and processes that shape our experiences and responses.

Role in Human Behaviour and Decision-Making

The subconscious mind plays a significant role in shaping human behaviour and decision-making processes in various ways:

1. Habit Formation: The subconscious mind is instrumental in forming habits. It stores repetitive actions and behaviours, allowing us to perform routine tasks without conscious effort.

2. Emotional Responses: Emotions are strongly tied to the subconscious. It processes and regulates emotions, impacting how we react to situations and people.

3. Memory Storage and Retrieval: The subconscious is a repository for memories. It stores experiences, learned behaviours, and information that influence our present actions and decisions. It also aids in memory retrieval, sometimes bringing forth information seemingly out of nowhere.

4. Influencing Choices: Subconscious beliefs, biases, and preferences often influence the decisions we make, even when we believe we are acting rationally. These hidden influences shape our preferences and guide our choices.

Historical Perspectives

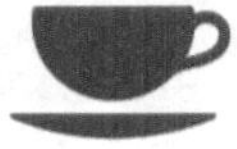

EVOLUTION OF THE CONCEPT of the Subconscious

The idea of the subconscious mind has a rich history that has evolved over centuries, shaping our understanding of human psychology and behaviour. The concept emerged from philosophical inquiries into the nature of the mind and gained prominence through influential theories proposed by key thinkers.

Ancient Roots and Philosophical Beginnings The exploration of the subconscious can be traced back to ancient philosophical traditions. Greek philosophers such as Plato and Aristotle contemplated the complexities of human consciousness, discussing the existence of unconscious mental processes. Plato's allegory of the cave and Aristotle's writings on dreams hinted at deeper layers of the mind beyond conscious awareness.

Early Modern Insights During the Renaissance and Enlightenment periods, discussions about the subconscious continued. René Descartes, with his dualistic view of mind and body, acknowledged the existence of mental processes that occur below conscious awareness. However, it was in the 19th and 20th centuries that the concept gained substantial attention and development.

Freudian Revolution: Sigmund Freud

Sigmund Freud, often regarded as the father of psychoanalysis, revolutionized the understanding of the subconscious. In the late 19th century, Freud proposed the idea of the unconscious mind, suggesting that hidden desires, traumatic experiences, and repressed thoughts significantly influence human behaviour. His psychoanalytic theories delved into the role of the unconscious in shaping personality, dreams, and mental disorders.

Freud's iceberg analogy, with the conscious mind as the tip and the subconscious and unconscious realms below the surface, visualized the layers of the mind and their relative accessibility to awareness.

Contributions of Carl Jung

Carl Jung, a contemporary of Freud and a renowned psychologist, expanded upon the concept of the unconscious. He introduced the notion of the collective unconscious, a deeper layer shared by all individuals that contains archetypes and universal symbols. Jung emphasized the importance of symbols, dreams, and myths in accessing and understanding the contents of the collective unconscious.

Influence on Modern Psychology

Freud and Jung's theories had a profound impact on psychology and laid the groundwork for further exploration into the subconscious. Their ideas sparked debates, criticism, and subsequent developments in psychoanalysis, cognitive psychology, and neuroscience.

Influential Theories and Thinkers

Apart from Freud and Jung, several other influential figures contributed to shaping our understanding of the subconscious:

William James

William James, an American philosopher and psychologist, explored the concepts of the subconscious and unconscious mental processes. He proposed the idea of the "stream of consciousness," highlighting the continuous flow of thoughts and perceptions, both conscious and unconscious.

Pierre Janet

Pierre Janet, a French psychologist, conducted extensive research on dissociation and subconscious processes. His work on trauma, dissociative disorders, and subconscious mechanisms influenced later psychological theories.

Contemporary Perspectives

Contemporary psychology continues to explore and refine the concept of the subconscious. Cognitive psychologists, behavioural scientists, and neuroscientists study implicit biases, automatic behaviours, and cognitive processes occurring below conscious awareness.

5. Problem Solving and Creativity: The subconscious mind is also involved in problem-solving and creative thinking. Sometimes, solutions to problems or creative ideas emerge seemingly from nowhere, a result of subconscious processing.

Understanding the subconscious mind's existence and its impact on human behaviour can lead to greater self-awareness. By recognizing and acknowledging these hidden influences, individuals can work towards making more informed and intentional decisions, thus gaining better control over their lives.

Conscious vs. Subconscious

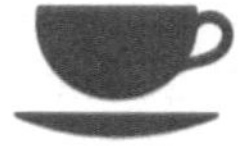

DIFFERENTIATING BETWEEN Conscious and Subconscious Processes

Conscious Mind

The conscious mind encompasses the thoughts, perceptions, sensations, and feelings that individuals are actively aware of at any given moment. It involves rational thinking, logical reasoning, and deliberate decision-making. When we're conscious, we're aware of our surroundings, thoughts, and actions in real-time.

Key Characteristics of the Conscious Mind:

1. Awareness: Consciousness involves being present and cognizant of one's immediate experiences.

2. Reasoning and Logic: It engages in critical thinking, problem-solving, and decision-making based on present information.

3. Limited Capacity: The conscious mind has limited capacity, and it's where short-term memories are stored temporarily.

Subconscious Mind

The subconscious mind operates below the level of conscious awareness. It contains a vast reservoir of information, memories, emotions, and automatic processes that influence thoughts, behaviours, and experiences without individuals actively realizing it. It functions beyond immediate awareness but significantly shapes our actions and perceptions.

Key Characteristics of the Subconscious Mind:

1. Automatic Processes: Subconscious processes are automatic and run in the background without conscious effort.

2. Emotional Centre: It strongly influences emotions, habits, and intuitive responses.

3. Vast Storage: The subconscious mind stores long-term memories, learned behaviours, beliefs, and conditioning.

Interaction and Influence on Behaviour

Coexistence and Integration

The conscious and subconscious minds work in tandem, continuously interacting and influencing each other. While the conscious mind engages in deliberate reasoning, the subconscious mind operates simultaneously, providing automatic responses and influencing perceptions.

Influence on Decision-Making

Behaviour and decision-making are often shaped by both conscious and subconscious processes:

- Conscious Influence: When making rational choices, individuals consider facts, logic, and immediate information within their conscious awareness.

- Subconscious Influence: Deep-seated beliefs, biases, emotions, and past experiences stored in the subconscious can subtly guide decisions, sometimes overriding conscious intentions.

Role in Habit Formation and Learning

The subconscious mind is instrumental in forming habits and learned behaviours. Through repetition and reinforcement, actions become automatic and stored in the subconscious. Even when consciously trying to change habits, the subconscious can resist alterations due to ingrained patterns.

Emotional Influence

Emotions strongly tie to the subconscious. Emotional responses often stem from subconscious processes, impacting behaviour without explicit conscious reasoning. The subconscious also stores emotional memories that can influence future reactions and decisions.

Harnessing the Interaction for Personal Growth

Understanding the interplay between the conscious and subconscious minds is essential for personal development:

- Self-Awareness: Recognizing subconscious influences allows for greater self-awareness, enabling individuals to understand their motivations and behaviours better.

- Mindfulness and Control: Mindfulness practices help bring subconscious processes into conscious awareness, allowing individuals to exert more control over their thoughts and reactions.

- Reprogramming Beliefs: By consciously challenging and reshaping subconscious beliefs, individuals can modify behaviours and achieve personal growth.

Formation and Function of the Subconscious Mind

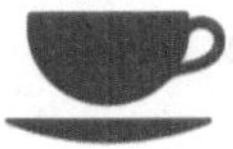

FORMATION OF THE SUBCONSCIOUS Mind

Early Developmental Stages

The subconscious mind begins its formation during early developmental stages, particularly in childhood. Experiences, interactions, and environmental influences play a crucial role in shaping the subconscious:

1. Early Impressions: Infants and young children absorb information from their surroundings, forming foundational beliefs and perceptions.

2. Family Dynamics: Family upbringing, parental interactions, and caregiver relationships deeply impact subconscious beliefs and emotional patterns.

3. Social Environment: Cultural norms, societal values, and peer interactions contribute to subconscious programming.

Encoding Memories and Experiences

The subconscious mind stores memories and experiences through various mechanisms:

1. Implicit Learning: Unconscious acquisition of knowledge and skills through repeated exposure and experiences.

2. Emotional Encoding: Emotional events and experiences are often strongly encoded in the subconscious, influencing future emotional responses.

3. Trauma and Conditioning: Traumatic experiences or intense conditioning can deeply impact

the subconscious, sometimes leading to long-lasting effects.

Belief Systems and Conditioning

Belief systems and conditioning significantly shape the subconscious mind:

1. Core Beliefs: Fundamental beliefs about oneself, the world, and others are ingrained in the subconscious, influencing perceptions and behaviours.

2. Conditioned Responses: Repetitive experiences and learned behaviours become automatic responses stored in the subconscious.

Functions and Mechanisms of the Subconscious Mind

Memory Storage and Retrieval

The subconscious mind serves as a reservoir for memories:

1. Long-Term Storage: It stores long-term memories, including past experiences, learned behaviours, and emotional imprints.

2. Memory Retrieval: Memories stored in the subconscious can resurface consciously or influence behaviour without explicit recall.

Automatic Processing and Habits

The subconscious operates in an automatic mode for various functions:

1. Habit Formation: It plays a crucial role in forming habits and routines, allowing for automatic execution of familiar tasks.

2. Automatic Behaviours: Subconscious processes govern various bodily functions, from breathing to complex motor skills, without conscious intervention.

Emotional Centre and Intuition

Emotions are deeply tied to the subconscious mind:

1. Emotional Processing: The subconscious influences emotional responses, shaping reactions and perceptions based on past emotional experiences.

2. Intuitive Insights: Subconscious processing sometimes provides intuitive insights or solutions to problems without conscious reasoning.

Influence on Decision-Making and Behaviour

The subconscious mind significantly impacts decision-making and behaviour:

1. Decision Influences: Hidden beliefs, biases, and emotional responses stored in the subconscious influence conscious choices and actions.

2. Behavioural Patterns: Learned behaviours and conditioned responses stored in the subconscious guide everyday actions, often without conscious awareness.

Neurobiological Mechanisms

The subconscious mind's functioning involves complex neurobiological processes:

1. Neural Networks: Specific neural pathways and connections facilitate subconscious processing and information retrieval.

2. Brain Structures: Regions like the amygdala, hippocampus, and prefrontal cortex play roles in subconscious functions, memory storage, and emotional regulation.

The subconscious mind forms through a combination of early developmental experiences, encoding of memories, belief systems, and conditioning. Its functions encompass memory storage, automatic processing, emotional regulation, and profound influence on decision-making and behaviour. Understanding the mechanisms behind subconscious functioning provides insight into how individuals perceive the world, make decisions, and behave, paving the way for potential interventions and personal development strategies.

Subconscious Processing: Role in Memory, Emotions, and Habits

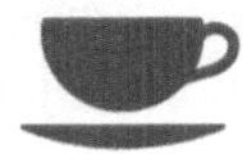

INFORMATION PROCESSING in the Subconscious
Encoding and Storage of Information
1. Implicit Learning: The subconscious mind constantly absorbs information implicitly, through repeated exposure and experiences, without conscious effort.

2. Selective Filtering: It filters and processes vast amounts of sensory information, selecting what is deemed relevant for storage and further processing.

3. Emotional Encoding: Emotions strongly influence how information is encoded and stored in the subconscious. Emotionally charged experiences tend to be more deeply imprinted.

Automatic Processing
1. Parallel Processing: The subconscious can handle multiple tasks simultaneously, processing information in parallel without overwhelming the conscious mind.

2. Efficiency in Routine Tasks: It efficiently manages routine actions and behaviours, freeing the conscious mind for more complex cognitive processes.

Role in Memory
Long-Term Memory Storage

1. Storage of Experiences: The subconscious mind stores a vast repository of memories, including experiences, learned behaviours, and associations, often inaccessible to immediate conscious recall.

2. Retrieval Mechanisms: Memories stored in the subconscious can resurface consciously, triggered by external cues or internal associations.

Implicit Memory

1. Implicit Memory Formation: It underpins implicit memory, where previous experiences influence current behaviour or thought patterns without conscious awareness of the initial experience.

2. Habitual Recall: Learned behaviours and skills become automated through repetition and are stored in the subconscious for quick retrieval.

Influence on Emotions

Emotional Regulation

1. Emotional Processing: The subconscious mind regulates emotional responses, drawing from stored emotional experiences to shape immediate reactions.

2. Emotionally Charged Decisions: Emotions stored in the subconscious influence decision-making and behaviours, sometimes overriding conscious reasoning.

Emotional Memory Association

1. Emotional Memories: Emotional experiences are often strongly linked to subconscious memory storage, impacting future emotional responses and perceptions.

2. Trauma and Emotional Imprints: Traumatic events can leave deep emotional imprints in the subconscious, affecting emotional well-being and behaviour.

Role in Habit Formation

Habitual Behaviour and Conditioning

1. Automatic Responses: The subconscious plays a pivotal role in forming habits by automating behaviours through repetition and reinforcement.

2. Resistance to Change: Ingrained habits and conditioned responses stored in the subconscious can resist conscious efforts to change behaviour.

Neural Pathways and Habit Formation

1. Neuroplasticity: The subconscious establishes neural pathways associated with repeated behaviours, making habits more entrenched over time.

2. Rewiring through Consistent Practice: Consistent conscious effort can gradually rewire subconscious neural pathways, leading to habit modification.

The subconscious mind processes information continually, encoding and storing experiences, emotions, and habits. Its role in memory involves the storage and retrieval of vast amounts of information, including implicit memories that influence behaviour without conscious awareness. Furthermore, the subconscious strongly influences emotional responses, regulating emotions based on stored experiences. Inhabit formation, it automates behaviours through repetition, forming neural pathways that guide automatic responses. Understanding the subconscious processing provides insight into how memories, emotions, and habits are formed and can be leveraged for personal growth and behavioural modifications.

Neurobiology of the Subconscious

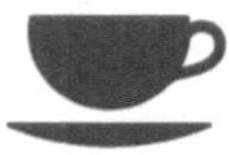

BRAIN STRUCTURES AND their Connection to the Subconscious
Amygdala
1. Emotional Processing: The amygdala, located in the temporal lobes, plays a pivotal role in emotional responses and emotional memory formation within the subconscious.
2. Fear and Anxiety: It's particularly associated with processing fear responses and emotional memories tied to fear-inducing stimuli.
Hippocampus
1. Memory Formation: The hippocampus, closely linked to the amygdala, aids in the formation and consolidation of explicit memories, playing a crucial role in transferring information to long-term memory in the subconscious.
2. Spatial Navigation: It contributes to spatial navigation and contextual memory, influencing how environmental cues are stored subconsciously.
Prefrontal Cortex
1. Executive Functions: The prefrontal cortex governs higher-order cognitive functions, overseeing decision-making, planning, and problem-solving, often in conjunction with the subconscious mind.
2. Integration with Subconscious: It interacts with deeper brain structures, modulating conscious

decision-making and influencing subconscious processes.

Neural Pathways Involved in Subconscious Processes

Basal Ganglia

1. Habit Formation: The basal ganglia, through its connection with the prefrontal cortex, plays a vital role in habit formation and procedural memory stored in the subconscious.

2. Automatic Motor Functions: It regulates automatic motor functions and skills, contributing to subconscious execution of learned behaviours.

Reticular Activating System (RAS)

1. Arousal and Attention: The RAS, located in the brainstem, regulates arousal and attention, filtering incoming sensory information and determining what reaches conscious awareness.

2. Influence on Alertness: It influences states of consciousness, guiding the attention of the conscious mind based on subconscious assessments.

Default Mode Network (DMN)

1. Self-Reflection and Memory Integration: The DMN, involving various brain regions like the medial prefrontal cortex and posterior cingulate cortex, is active during rest and self-reflection.

2. Memory Consolidation: It aids in integrating information from the conscious and subconscious, contributing to memory consolidation processes.

Thalamus

1. Sensory Relay Centre: The thalamus serves as a relay centre for sensory information, directing it to various brain regions for further processing.

2. Gatekeeper of Consciousness: It filters sensory input, allowing only a fraction to reach conscious awareness while influencing subconscious processing.

The subconscious mind's neurobiology involves a complex interplay of various brain structures and neural pathways. Regions like the amygdala and hippocampus are critical for emotional processing and memory formation within the subconscious. Additionally, the prefrontal cortex modulates higher cognitive functions and integrates with deeper brain structures, influencing subconscious processes. Neural pathways like the basal ganglia and RAS play pivotal roles in habit formation, attention regulation, and filtering sensory input, shaping subconscious and conscious experiences. Understanding the neurobiological underpinnings of the subconscious sheds light on how brain structures and pathways collaborate to process information, form memories, and guide behaviour beyond conscious awareness.

Subconscious Influence on Behaviour

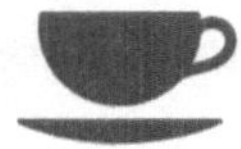

THE SUBCONSCIOUS MIND exerts a profound influence on human behaviour, playing a pivotal role in decision-making, habit formation, and shaping perceptions. Understanding how subconscious thoughts affect behaviour unveils the intricate mechanisms guiding our actions beyond conscious awareness.

Impact on Decision-Making

Hidden Biases and Beliefs

1. Implicit Biases: Subconscious biases, often rooted in societal conditioning or personal experiences, impact decision-making without conscious acknowledgment.

2. Cultural and Social Influence: Subconscious beliefs assimilated from cultural norms and societal expectations subtly steer choices and judgments.

Emotional Influences

1. Emotional Responses: Subconscious emotions greatly impact decision-making, sometimes leading to choices based on past emotional imprints stored in the subconscious.

2. Intuitive Decisions: Gut feelings or intuitive decisions often stem from subconscious processing, guiding choices based on feelings rather than conscious reasoning.

Subconscious Processing of Information

1. Information Integration: The subconscious mind integrates vast amounts of information beyond conscious capacity, influencing decisions based on accumulated data.

2. Pattern Recognition: It recognizes patterns and associations derived from stored experiences, guiding decision-making through implicit learning.

Role in Habit Formation

Automatic Behavioural Responses

1. Habitual Actions: Subconscious thoughts reinforce habitual behaviours, shaping daily routines and automatic responses to stimuli without conscious intervention.

2. Resistance to Change: Efforts to alter habits often face resistance from the subconscious, as ingrained behaviours are deeply rooted.

Neural Pathways and Reinforcement

1. Neurological Changes: Subconscious thoughts form neural pathways through repetition, reinforcing behaviours and making them more automatic.

2. Reward-Based Learning: The subconscious seeks familiar and rewarding patterns, reinforcing behaviours associated with pleasurable outcomes.

Influence on Perceptions

Shaping Worldview

1. Perceptual Filters: Subconscious beliefs act as filters, shaping how individuals perceive the world and interpret incoming information.

2. Confirmation Bias: Subconscious thoughts often lead to selective attention, favouring information that aligns with existing beliefs and disregarding contradictory evidence.

Emotional Lens

1. Emotion-Driven Perceptions: Subconscious emotions colour perceptions, influencing how situations and people are interpreted and responded to.

2. Emotional Memories: Past emotional experiences stored in the subconscious shape perceptions and affect present reactions.

Managing Subconscious Influence

Increased Self-Awareness

1. Recognizing Patterns: Understanding subconscious influences fosters self-awareness, allowing individuals to recognize recurring patterns in behaviour and decisions.

2. Mindfulness Practices: Mindfulness aids in bringing subconscious thoughts to conscious awareness, enabling better control over behavioural responses.

Intentional Reprogramming

1. Challenging Beliefs: Actively challenging and reshaping subconscious beliefs can lead to behaviour modification and a shift in decision-making processes.

2. Visualization and Affirmations: Techniques like visualization and positive affirmations reprogram subconscious thoughts, fostering a more empowering mindset.

The subconscious mind profoundly shapes human behaviour by influencing decision-making processes, habit formation, and perceptions. Its impact extends beyond conscious awareness, steering actions based on hidden biases, emotions, and learned behaviours. Understanding the subconscious influence on behaviour empowers individuals to cultivate greater

self-awareness, enabling intentional reprogramming
of beliefs and behaviours for personal growth and
enhanced decision-making. Recognizing and
managing subconscious thoughts can lead to more
informed and intentional choices, fostering positive
changes in behaviour and perceptions.

Emotions and the Subconscious

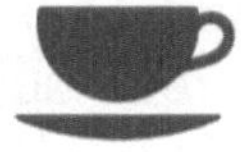

THE INTERPLAY BETWEEN emotions and the subconscious mind is intricate, influencing how individuals perceive, process, and respond to emotional stimuli. Understanding the role of the subconscious in emotional responses and regulation unveils the mechanisms that shape our emotional experiences.

Subconscious Influence on Emotional Responses

Emotional Memory Processing

1. Storage of Emotional Experiences: The subconscious mind stores emotional memories, influencing immediate emotional reactions to similar situations.

2. Impact of Past Trauma: Traumatic experiences stored in the subconscious may trigger intense emotional responses without conscious control.

Implicit Emotional Associations

1. Associative Learning: Subconscious thoughts link emotions to specific stimuli or experiences, affecting emotional responses without conscious awareness of the association.

2. Implicit Emotional Triggers: Triggers from subconscious associations prompt emotional reactions, often bypassing conscious reasoning.

Intuitive Emotional Reactions

1. Subconscious Intuition: The subconscious provides intuitive insights based on emotional cues,

guiding decisions and behaviours through instinctual emotional responses.

2. Gut Feelings and Hunches: Gut feelings or hunches often arise from subconscious emotional processing, guiding individuals without explicit conscious reasoning.

Processing and Regulation of Emotions

Emotional Processing

1. Emotional Filtering and Assessment: The subconscious evaluates incoming emotional information, filtering and assigning significance to various stimuli.

2. Emotional Integration: It integrates emotional experiences into memory, influencing future emotional responses and perceptions.

Emotional Regulation

1. Automatic Emotional Regulation: The subconscious regulates emotions based on stored experiences, attempting to maintain emotional balance without conscious effort.

2. Emotion Suppression or Repression: In some cases, the subconscious suppresses or represses intense emotions, affecting conscious emotional experiences.

Influence of Subconscious in Emotional Health

Emotional Resilience and Coping Mechanisms

1. Adaptive Coping Strategies: Subconscious thoughts influence the development of coping mechanisms and resilience strategies to navigate emotional challenges.

2. Influence on Emotional Well-being: Deep-seated beliefs stored in the subconscious shape

emotional responses, impacting overall emotional health.

Emotional Expression and Communication

1. Unconscious Communication: Subconscious emotional cues, such as body language and facial expressions, play a role in non-verbal emotional communication.

2. Impact on Interpersonal Dynamics: Unconscious emotional signals influence interpersonal relationships, affecting how emotions are perceived and reciprocated.

Managing Subconscious Influence on Emotions

Self-Awareness and Emotional Insight

1. Recognizing Emotional Triggers: Understanding subconscious emotional triggers aids in identifying patterns and managing emotional reactions more effectively.

2. Emotional Self-Reflection: Reflecting on subconscious emotional processes fosters self-awareness, enabling better emotional regulation.

Mindfulness and Emotional Regulation Techniques

1. Mindfulness Practices: Mindfulness cultivates awareness of present emotions, allowing individuals to acknowledge and manage subconscious emotional responses.

2. Emotion Regulation Strategies: Techniques like deep breathing, meditation, and cognitive reappraisal help regulate emotions influenced by subconscious thoughts.

The subconscious mind significantly shapes emotional responses, processing emotional experiences and regulating reactions beyond conscious control. It stores emotional memories, associates' emotions with specific triggers, and plays a pivotal role in intuitive emotional responses. Understanding the influence of the subconscious on emotions empowers individuals to develop greater emotional self-awareness and employ strategies for managing subconscious emotional triggers. Techniques like mindfulness and emotion regulation methods aid in navigating emotional experiences influenced by subconscious thoughts, fostering emotional resilience and well-being. Recognizing the interplay between emotions and the subconscious offers insights into emotional processing and the potential for intentional emotional regulation and growth.

Subconscious Learning and Conditioning

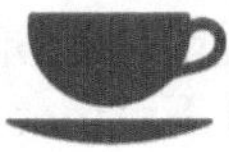

THE SUBCONSCIOUS MIND plays a pivotal role in learning and adaptation, incorporating experiences and environmental stimuli through various processes. Pavlovian (classical) and Skinnerian (operant) conditioning are prominent theories that illustrate how the subconscious learns, adapts, and forms behavioural responses.

Subconscious Learning Mechanisms

Implicit Learning

1. Unconscious Acquisition: Implicit learning occurs without deliberate intent or conscious awareness, allowing the subconscious to absorb information and patterns effortlessly.

2. Skill Acquisition: Subconscious learning enables the mastery of skills and behaviours through repeated exposure and practice.

Associative Learning

1. Linking Stimuli and Responses: The subconscious forms associations between stimuli and responses, influencing future reactions based on prior experiences.

2. Classical and Operant Conditioning: Associative learning forms the foundation of conditioning theories, shaping behavioural responses.

Pavlovian (Classical) Conditioning

Principles of Pavlovian Conditioning

1. Conditional Stimulus-Response Association: Pavlov's experiments demonstrated the formation of associations between a neutral stimulus (bell) and an unconditioned stimulus (food), leading to a conditioned response (salivation).

2. Acquisition and Extinction: The subconscious learns to associate stimuli, and extinction occurs when the conditioned response diminishes after the absence of the unconditioned stimulus.

Real-Life Applications

1. Phobias and Emotional Responses: Pavlovian conditioning underpins the development of phobias, where neutral stimuli become associated with fear responses.

2. Advertising and Branding: Marketers utilize associative techniques to create positive associations between products and desirable emotions, influencing consumer behaviour subconsciously.

Skinnerian (Operant) Conditioning

Principles of Operant Conditioning

1. Behaviour-Consequence Association: Skinner's theory emphasizes the relationship between behaviour and its consequences (reinforcement or punishment), shaping future behavioural responses.

2. Reinforcement Schedules: Different reinforcement schedules (e.g., fixed interval, variable ratio) influence the rate and consistency of subconscious learning.

Real-Life Applications

1. Behaviour Modification: Operant conditioning principles are employed in education, therapy, and organizational settings to modify behaviour through reinforcement strategies.

2. Reward Systems in Workplaces: Workplace environments often utilize reinforcement techniques, such as rewards or incentives, to shape employee behaviour subconsciously.

Subconscious Adaptation and Behavioural Changes

Habit Formation and Automatic Responses

1. Repetitive Conditioning: Subconscious learning leads to habitual behaviours, making actions automatic and requiring minimal conscious effort.

2. Resistance to Change: Ingrained behaviours conditioned in the subconscious may resist modification, requiring deliberate efforts to alter them.

Neuroplasticity and Subconscious Learning

1. Neural Rewiring: Subconscious learning triggers changes in neural pathways, allowing the brain to adapt and rewire based on new experiences and conditioning.

2. Age and Learning: While neuroplasticity declines with age, the subconscious can still adapt and learn, albeit at different rates.

The subconscious mind engages in various forms of learning and adaptation, shaping behavioural responses through mechanisms like implicit learning and associative processes. Pavlovian and Skinnerian conditioning theories elucidate how subconscious associations influence behaviour, leading to conditioned responses based on prior experiences and reinforcement. Understanding these subconscious learning mechanisms offers insights into how behaviours are acquired, reinforced, and modified, facilitating applications in diverse fields such as education, therapy, marketing, and behavioural modification strategies. Recognizing the subconscious's role in learning and conditioning empowers individuals and organizations to leverage these mechanisms for positive behavioural changes and adaptive learning.

Dreams and the Unconscious

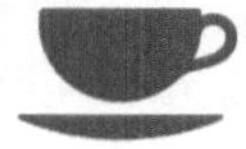

DREAMS SERVE AS A WINDOW into the subconscious mind, offering insights into emotions, desires, fears, and unresolved conflicts. Understanding the relationship between dreams and the subconscious involves exploring their interpretation, significance, and the connections they establish between the conscious and unconscious realms.

Understanding Dreams and their Link to the Subconscious

Nature of Dreams

1. Symbolic Representation: Dreams often communicate subconscious thoughts and emotions symbolically rather than in a literal manner.

2. Mixed Content: Dreams may encompass various elements, including personal experiences, fears, desires, memories, and random imagery.

The Unconscious in Dreams

1. Unconscious Expression: Dreams provide a platform for the unconscious mind to express repressed emotions, desires, and unresolved issues.

2. Subconscious Processing: Dream content reflects ongoing subconscious processing, integrating experiences and emotions into symbolic narratives.

Interpretation of Dreams

Symbolism and Metaphor

1. Dream Symbols: Objects, people, and scenarios in dreams often symbolize deeper subconscious

meanings rather than representing their literal counterparts.

2. Personal Associations: Interpretations consider personal associations and cultural symbolism, as dream symbols may vary in meaning for different individuals.

Analysing Dream Elements

1. Dream Themes: Identifying recurring themes or patterns in dreams assists in understanding persistent subconscious concerns or desires.

2. Emotional Tone: Examining the emotional tone of dreams aids in gauging underlying emotions and their significance.

Significance of Dreams

Emotional Processing and Resolution

1. Emotional Release: Dreams provide an avenue for emotional release, allowing the subconscious to process unresolved emotions or experiences.

2. Problem Solving: Some theories suggest that dreams aid in problem-solving, as the subconscious mind explores solutions or alternatives during sleep.

Self-Exploration and Insight

1. Self-Reflection: Dreams offer opportunities for self-reflection, enabling individuals to gain insights into their subconscious thoughts, conflicts, and desires.

2. Unconscious Awareness: Dreams may reveal aspects of the self that are not readily acknowledged or recognized in waking life.

Psychoanalytic Perspectives

Freudian Dream Analysis

1. Manifest and Latent Content: Freud proposed the division of dreams into manifest (surface) content

and latent (hidden) content, where the latter represents the true underlying meaning.

2. Wish Fulfilment: Freudian theory posits that dreams fulfil unconscious wishes, expressing repressed desires and conflicts in symbolic form.

Jungian Dream Interpretation

1. Archetypal Symbols: Carl Jung emphasized the role of archetypes in dreams, suggesting that dreams tap into collective symbols and universal themes.

2. Integration and Individuation: Jung viewed dreams as facilitating the integration of the conscious and unconscious aspects of the self, leading to individuation and personal growth.

Application and Personal Reflection

Dream Journaling and Analysis

1. Keeping a Dream Journal: Recording dreams enhances awareness of recurring themes and emotions, aiding in their interpretation and understanding.

2. Personal Growth: Reflecting on dream content facilitates self-exploration and personal development by integrating subconscious insights into waking life.

Therapeutic Use of Dreams

1. Dream Work in Therapy: Therapists employ dream analysis to uncover unconscious conflicts, aiding in the therapeutic process and promoting self-awareness.

2. Integration in Treatment: Understanding dreams contributes to addressing psychological issues and promoting emotional healing in therapeutic settings.

Dreams offer a unique pathway to explore the subconscious mind, providing symbolic representations of emotions, conflicts, desires, and unresolved issues. Interpreting dreams involves deciphering symbolic elements and analysing their significance in relation to an individual's experiences and emotions. The significance of dreams lies in their potential to facilitate emotional processing, problem-solving, self-exploration, and personal growth. Psychoanalytic perspectives from Freud and Jung offer frameworks to understand dreams' latent meanings and their relevance to the psyche. Engaging with dreams through journaling, analysis, and therapeutic exploration contributes to self-awareness, introspection, and potential psychological healing. Recognizing the connection between dreams and the subconscious fosters a deeper understanding of the hidden realms of the mind, unveiling insights that can enrich waking life and aid in personal development.

Freudian Analysis: The Unconscious and the Structure of the Mind

SIGMUND FREUD, THE founder of psychoanalysis, introduced revolutionary theories that delved into the depths of the unconscious mind and proposed a complex structure of the psyche comprising the id, ego, and superego. His theories profoundly influenced our understanding of human behaviour and the intricate workings of the mind.

Freud's Theories on the Unconscious

Unconscious Mind

1. Hidden Motivations and Desires: Freud posited that the unconscious mind contains repressed thoughts, memories, and desires that influence conscious behaviour.

2. Dynamic and Influential: The unconscious exerts powerful influence on thoughts, emotions, and behaviours, often beyond conscious awareness.

Unconscious Processes

1. Défense Mechanisms: Freud described defence mechanisms like repression, denial, and projection as ways the unconscious mind protects itself from anxiety-provoking thoughts or emotions.

2. Symbolic Representations: Dreams, slips of the tongue (Freudian slips), and humour were seen as avenues through which the unconscious expressed its hidden contents.

The Structure of the Mind: Id, Ego, and Superego
Id
1. Pleasure Principle: The id operates on the pleasure principle, seeking immediate gratification of primal urges, desires, and instincts.

2. Unconscious and Impulsive: It resides entirely in the unconscious and lacks rationality, driven by instincts such as hunger, aggression, and sexual impulses.

Ego
1. Reality Principle: The ego mediates between the id's impulses, the external world, and internalized societal norms, aiming for realistic and socially acceptable outcomes.

2. Conscious and Rational: The ego operates in the conscious and preconscious realms, employing rationality and problem-solving to navigate conflicting demands.

Superego
1. Internalized Morality: The superego represents societal and parental values, morality, and ethical standards internalized by an individual.

2. Conscience and Ego Ideal: It comprises the conscience (imposing moral standards) and the ego ideal (aspirational self-standards), guiding behaviour through guilt and pride.

Interplay among Id, Ego, and Superego
Conflict and Resolution
1. Intrapsychic Conflict: Freud proposed that conflicts arise between the id's desires, the superego's moral demands, and the ego's need to reconcile both, leading to anxiety.

2. Défense Mechanisms: The ego employs defence mechanisms to manage conflicts and reduce anxiety by distorting reality or repressing unacceptable impulses.

Criticisms and Contemporary Views

Criticisms of Freudian Theory

1. Lack of Empirical Evidence: Freud's theories faced criticism for their lack of empirical validation and reliance on subjective interpretations.

2. Gender and Cultural Biases: Critics pointed out biases in Freud's theories, particularly regarding gender and cultural generalizations.

Contemporary Relevance

1. Influence on Psychology: Despite criticisms, Freud's ideas laid the groundwork for psychoanalytic and psychodynamic approaches in psychology, influencing therapeutic practices.

2. Modified Concepts: Contemporary psychology has adapted and modified Freud's concepts, integrating them with empirical research and other psychological theories.

Freud's theories on the unconscious mind, as well as the id, ego, and superego, revolutionized our understanding of human psychology. His exploration of the unconscious and its impact on behaviour introduced concepts that continue to influence psychological thought. The id's primal drives, the ego's mediation, and the superego's moral standards form a dynamic interplay shaping human behaviour and personality. While Freud's theories faced criticism, they remain significant in the history of psychology, contributing to the development of various therapeutic approaches and our understanding of the complexities of the human mind. Contemporary psychology continues to build upon Freud's ideas, integrating them with empirical research and diverse perspectives, further evolving our understanding of the unconscious and the structures of the mind.

Jungian Archetypes: Carl Jung's Collective Unconscious

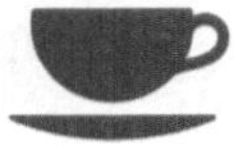

CARL JUNG, A PROMINENT figure in psychology, introduced the concept of the collective unconscious, proposing that the human psyche harbours universal symbols and patterns called archetypes. These archetypes are fundamental to Jung's theory, influencing human behaviour, thoughts, and experiences in profound ways.

The Collective Unconscious

Definition and Nature

1. Inherited Psychic Content: Jung conceptualized the collective unconscious as a reservoir of inherited, universal, and symbolic content shared by all humans.

2. Beyond Personal Experience: It comprises themes, symbols, and archetypes that transcend individual experiences and are common across cultures and times.

Archetypes

1. Archetypal Patterns: Archetypes are universal, instinctive patterns or symbols residing within the collective unconscious, representing fundamental human themes.

2. Symbolic Representations: They manifest as characters, motifs, or themes in myths, folklore, dreams, and cultural narratives.

Types of Archetypes

Persona

1. Social Mask: The persona represents the social identity or mask individuals present to the world, shaped by societal expectations and norms.

2. Adaptation and Social Integration: It facilitates social interaction and adaptation but may conceal deeper aspects of the self.

Shadow

1. Repressed and Unacknowledged Aspects: The shadow embodies the hidden, repressed, or rejected aspects of the self, often containing dark, unacknowledged desires, fears, or traits.

2. Integration and Personal Growth: Integrating the shadow involves acknowledging and reconciling with these aspects, leading to personal growth and self-awareness.

Anima/Animus

1. Feminine and Masculine Aspects: Anima represents the feminine aspects within the male psyche, while animus represents the masculine aspects within the female psyche.

2. Integration and Wholeness: Developing a balanced relationship with the anima/animus fosters inner harmony and wholeness, transcending gender roles.

Self

1. Wholeness and Integration: The self represents the totality of the psyche, aiming for balance and integration of all aspects, including conscious and unconscious elements.

2. Individuation Process: Individuation involves aligning with the self, achieving personal growth, and realizing one's unique potential.

Influence of Archetypes

Symbolic Expression

1. Dreams and Myths: Archetypes manifest in dreams, fantasies, and cultural narratives, expressing universal themes and symbolizing human experiences.

2. Art, Literature, and Religion: Artists, writers, and religious symbols often draw upon archetypal themes, resonating with collective human experiences.

Psychological Development

1. Personal Transformation: Engaging with archetypes supports psychological development, fostering self-discovery, and promoting individuation.

2. Guiding Life Transitions: Archetypes offer guidance during life transitions and crises, aiding individuals in navigating challenges and transformations.

Criticisms and Contemporary Views

Criticisms of Jung's Theory

1. Lack of Empirical Evidence: Jung's ideas on archetypes lack empirical support, raising questions about their scientific validity.

2. Overemphasizing Unconscious Influence: Critics argue that Jung may have overemphasized the influence of the unconscious and symbolic representations.

Contemporary Relevance

1. Integration in Depth Psychology: Despite criticisms, Jung's concepts continue to influence depth psychology, psychotherapy, and cultural studies.

2. Integration with Modern Psychology: Contemporary psychology integrates elements of

Jungian theory with empirical research, exploring connections between symbolism and cognition.

Carl Jung's theory of the collective unconscious and archetypes revolutionized psychology by highlighting the universality of symbolic representations within the human psyche. Archetypes, such as the persona, shadow, anima/animus, and self, serve as symbolic patterns guiding human experiences and personal development. They manifest in dreams, myths, art, and cultural narratives, expressing fundamental human themes and facilitating psychological growth. While Jung's theories face criticism for their lack of empirical evidence, they remain influential in-depth psychology, psychotherapy, and cultural studies. Contemporary psychology continues to explore and integrate elements of Jungian theory, bridging symbolic representations with empirical research, furthering our understanding of the depths of the human psyche and the influence of archetypes on human behaviour and development.

Harnessing the Power of the Subconscious Mind

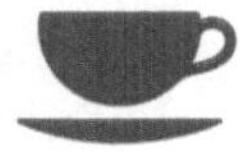

THE SUBCONSCIOUS MIND possesses immense potential, influencing our thoughts, behaviours, and perceptions. Various techniques allow individuals to access and harness the power of the subconscious, including visualization, affirmations, and meditation. These methods aim to tap into the subconscious to promote personal growth, enhance well-being, and facilitate positive change.

Visualization Techniques

Mental Imagery

1. Creating Mental Pictures: Visualization involves creating vivid mental images or scenarios to stimulate the subconscious mind.

2. Positive Visualization: Envisioning desired outcomes or goals engages the subconscious, influencing attitudes and actions toward achieving those objectives.

Guided Imagery

1. Directed Visualization: Guided imagery employs recorded scripts or instructions to guide individuals through detailed mental scenarios, often used in relaxation or therapeutic settings.

2. Targeted Emotional Responses: By visualizing calming or positive experiences, individuals can influence emotions and reduce stress or anxiety.

Affirmations and Positive Suggestions

Power of Affirmations

1. Positive Self-Talk: Affirmations involve repeating positive statements to instil belief in one's abilities or desired outcomes.

2. Reprogramming the Subconscious: Affirmations help counter negative self-talk and reshape subconscious beliefs by reinforcing positive messages.

Effective Affirmation Practices

1. Present-Tense Statements: Crafting affirmations in the present tense reinforces the belief that desired outcomes are already happening or achievable.

2. Consistent Repetition: Regular repetition of affirmations enhances their impact, gradually influencing subconscious thoughts and attitudes.

Meditation Practices

Mindfulness Meditation

1. Focused Awareness: Mindfulness meditation involves maintaining present-moment awareness, observing thoughts and sensations without judgment.

2. Calming the Mind: By quieting mental chatter, mindfulness allows individuals to access deeper layers of the subconscious and foster clarity.

Transcendental Meditation

1. Mantra-based Practice: Transcendental meditation uses repeated silent mantras to facilitate relaxation and access deeper states of consciousness.

2. Stress Reduction and Self-Exploration: It promotes relaxation and self-reflection, aiding in stress reduction and exploring subconscious thoughts and experiences.

Hypnotherapy and Self-Hypnosis

Inducing Altered States

1. Focused Attention: Hypnotherapy involves inducing a trance-like state, enhancing focus, and increasing suggestibility to access the subconscious.

2. Self-Suggestions and Behaviour Modification: Self-hypnosis techniques allow individuals to apply suggestions for behaviour modification or self-improvement.

Clinical and Therapeutic Applications

1. Addressing Psychological Issues: Hypnotherapy is used to explore and address subconscious issues, traumas, or habits contributing to psychological concerns.

2. Pain Management and Relaxation: It aids in pain management, stress reduction, and promoting relaxation by accessing deeper states of the mind.

Integration and Best Practices

Combined Techniques

1. Synergy of Methods: Combining visualization, affirmations, meditation, and hypnosis amplifies their impact, accessing different facets of the subconscious.

2. Consistent Practice: Regularity and commitment to these practices yield better results, reinforcing positive changes in the subconscious mind over time.

Ethical Considerations

1. Self-Responsibility: Practitioners should approach subconscious techniques responsibly, ensuring alignment with personal values and ethical considerations.

2. Professional Guidance: Seeking guidance from qualified practitioners or therapists is advisable, especially when addressing deep-seated issues or traumas.

Accessing and utilizing the power of the subconscious mind through techniques like visualization, affirmations, meditation, and hypnotherapy offer pathways to personal growth, well-being, and behavioural change. These practices engage the subconscious, allowing individuals to reprogram beliefs, reduce stress, manage emotions, and explore deeper aspects of the psyche. Consistent practice and ethical considerations are crucial for effectively harnessing the subconscious, promoting positive changes, and unlocking the immense potential within the depths of the mind.

Reprogramming Subconscious Beliefs

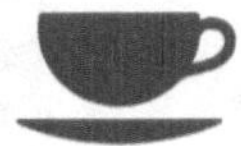

OVERCOMING LIMITING Patterns

The subconscious mind operates based on beliefs and thought patterns acquired over time, often influencing behaviour, emotions, and perceptions. Reprogramming these subconscious beliefs involves techniques aimed at identifying, challenging, and replacing limiting beliefs and negative thought patterns with more empowering ones. Through targeted practices and strategies, individuals can initiate positive changes and foster a more supportive subconscious environment.

Identifying Limiting Beliefs

Self-Reflection and Awareness

1. Examining Core Beliefs: Reflecting on recurring patterns or beliefs that hinder personal growth and well-being.

2. Tracing Emotional Responses: Noticing emotional reactions to situations can indicate underlying beliefs influencing responses.

Journaling and Self-Examination

1. Recording Thoughts and Reactions: Maintaining a journal to track thoughts, emotions, and situations linked to limiting beliefs.

2. Questioning Assumptions: Engaging in self-inquiry to challenge the validity of beliefs and their origins.

Challenging Negative Thought Patterns

Cognitive Restructuring

1. Examining Evidence: Assessing the evidence supporting or refuting negative beliefs, encouraging a more balanced perspective.

2. Alternative Interpretations: Identifying alternative explanations for situations, allowing for more constructive interpretations.

Reframing Techniques

1. Positive Reframing: Transforming negative thoughts into positive or neutral ones, altering the emotional impact of situations.

2. Language Adjustment: Choosing empowering language and internal dialogue to cultivate supportive beliefs.

Affirmations and Positive Reinforcement

Crafting Empowering Affirmations

1. Specific and Present-Tense Statements: Creating affirmations that directly counteract limiting beliefs, reinforcing positive messages in the present tense.

2. Consistent Repetition: Regularly repeating affirmations to reinforce new beliefs and counteract negative thought patterns.

Visualization and Imagery

1. Visualizing Success and Growth: Engaging in mental imagery to vividly picture desired outcomes, encouraging the subconscious to align with positive visions.

2. Emotional Engagement: Involving emotions during visualization enhances the impact on subconscious reprogramming.

Neuro-Linguistic Programming (NLP) Techniques

Anchoring and Pattern Interruption

1. Anchoring Positive States: Linking empowering emotions to specific triggers or actions, establishing positive anchors for subconscious responses.

2. Interrupting Negative Cycles: Identifying habitual negative thought patterns and interrupting them by introducing new, positive behaviours or thoughts.

Modelling and Behaviour Observation

1. Modelling Success: Observing and learning from individuals who exhibit the desired traits or behaviours, aiding in adopting new patterns at a subconscious level.

2. Behavioural Replication: Emulating successful behaviours gradually integrates them into one's own subconscious repertoire.

Meditation and Mindfulness Practices

Mindfulness-Based Cognitive Therapy

1. Observing Thoughts Non-Judgmentally: Mindfulness practices allow individuals to observe thoughts without attachment or judgment, reducing the impact of negative beliefs.

2. Acceptance and Detachment: Cultivating a sense of detachment from negative thoughts fosters a more objective perspective.

Affirmative Meditation

1. Affirmation Integration: Combining meditation practices with affirmations or positive visualizations reinforces their impact on the subconscious.

2. State of Relaxation: Meditative states relax the mind, making it more receptive to reprogramming efforts.

Integration and Consistency

Commitment to Practice

1. Consistency in Techniques: Regular and committed practice of reprogramming techniques enhances their effectiveness in altering subconscious beliefs.

2. Integration into Daily Routine: Incorporating reprogramming exercises into daily habits aids in sustaining efforts and reinforcing positive changes.

Patience and Persistence

1. Gradual Progression: Acknowledging that changing deep-seated beliefs takes time and persistence, avoiding discouragement from slow progress.

2. Celebrating Small Wins: Recognizing and celebrating even minor shifts in beliefs encourages further motivation and dedication.

Reprogramming subconscious beliefs involves a multifaceted approach encompassing awareness, challenging negative patterns, and introducing empowering techniques. By actively engaging in practices like cognitive restructuring, affirmations, visualization, and mindfulness, individuals can identify, confront, and replace limiting beliefs with more empowering ones. Consistency, commitment, and patience are essential in this journey, as gradual but persistent efforts yield significant changes in reshaping the subconscious landscape. Integrating these techniques into daily life promotes lasting transformation, fostering a more supportive and empowering subconscious environment conducive to personal growth and well-being.

The Subconscious in Various Therapeutic Approaches

The subconscious mind plays a crucial role in numerous therapeutic modalities, influencing the effectiveness of treatments and facilitating psychological healing. Understanding the interplay between the subconscious and different therapeutic approaches, such as Cognitive Behavioural Therapy (CBT), hypnotherapy, and psychoanalysis, sheds light on how these techniques harness subconscious processes to promote mental health and well-being.

Cognitive Behavioural Therapy (CBT)

Conscious-Restructuring Techniques

1. Identifying Cognitive Distortions: CBT involves recognizing and challenging negative thought patterns and beliefs that influence emotions and behaviours.

2. Conscious Thought Modification: Clients learn to reframe negative thoughts consciously, altering their impact on emotions and actions.

Subconscious Influence

1. Automatic Thoughts: Unconscious beliefs influence automatic thoughts targeted in CBT sessions, impacting emotional responses and behaviours.

2. Root Beliefs Exploration: Exploring underlying beliefs, often originating in the subconscious, aids in addressing core issues affecting thoughts and behaviours.

Hypnotherapy

Accessing the Subconscious

1. Inducing Trance States: Hypnotherapy aims to access the subconscious through trance-like states,

enhancing suggestibility and accessing deeper layers of the mind.

2. Subconscious Suggestions: Therapists deliver positive suggestions to the subconscious, targeting behaviour modification or addressing deep-seated issues.

Uncovering Subconscious Content

1. Regressing to Root Causes: Regression techniques in hypnotherapy access subconscious memories or experiences influencing current behaviours or beliefs.

2. Resolving Trauma and Phobias: Exploring and processing subconscious content aids in resolving traumatic experiences or phobic reactions.

Psychoanalytic and Psychodynamic Therapy

Exploring the Unconscious

1. Free Association and Dream Analysis: Techniques involve exploring free associations and dreams, accessing unconscious thoughts, emotions, and conflicts.

2. Transference and Countertransference: Unconscious projections and dynamics in the therapeutic relationship reveal subconscious patterns and unresolved issues.

Unconscious Conflict Resolution

1. Working through Resistance: Identifying and addressing resistance in therapy often reveals underlying subconscious conflicts or defences.

2. Interpreting Symbolism: Analysing symbols and patterns in client narratives aids in understanding subconscious content and unresolved issues.

Gestalt Therapy

Embracing Subconscious Expression

1. Experiential Techniques: Gestalt therapy focuses on present experiences, including bodily sensations and emotions, often rooted in the subconscious.

2. Empty Chair Technique: Encouraging dialogue with parts of the self-reveals subconscious conflicts and facilitates resolution.

Integrating the Unconscious

1. Heightening Awareness: Techniques focus on increasing awareness of subconscious processes, integrating fragmented aspects of the self.

2. Symbolic Exploration: Gestalt therapy utilizes symbols and metaphors, exploring their meaning and connections to the subconscious.

Acceptance and Commitment Therapy (ACT)

Mindfulness and Subconscious Processes

1. Mindfulness Practices: ACT incorporates mindfulness techniques to observe thoughts and emotions, fostering awareness of subconscious processes.

2. Diffusion Techniques: Disentangling from negative thoughts reduces their impact on behaviour, addressing subconscious influences.

Values and Subconscious Alignment

1. Clarifying Values: ACT helps individuals identify core values, aligning behaviours and goals with subconscious beliefs and aspirations.

2. Psychological Flexibility: Embracing thoughts and feelings facilitates psychological flexibility, integrating subconscious elements with conscious actions.

Integrative and Holistic Approaches

Multimodal Techniques

1. Blending Therapeutic Approaches: Integrative therapies combine methods from various modalities to address subconscious, cognitive, emotional, and behavioural aspects.

2. Holistic Healing: Approaches like mindfulness-based interventions or body-oriented therapies incorporate subconscious influences for comprehensive healing.

Subconscious Integration

1. Body-Mind Connection: Techniques that explore body sensations or somatic experiences connect subconscious processes with physical sensations and emotions.

2. Narrative and Expressive Therapies: Using creative mediums allows subconscious expression through storytelling, art, or movement.

Therapeutic approaches vary in their methods but converge in their recognition of the subconscious's pivotal role in influencing thoughts, emotions, and behaviours. Cognitive Behavioural Therapy targets conscious thoughts and behaviours influenced by underlying subconscious beliefs. Hypnotherapy, psychoanalytic therapy, and Gestalt therapy delve deeper, accessing and addressing subconscious content directly. Approaches like ACT and integrative therapies incorporate mindfulness and holistic elements, recognizing the importance of subconscious processes in fostering psychological well-being. Understanding the interaction between the subconscious and therapeutic techniques guides clinicians in tailoring interventions to access and address underlying beliefs and patterns, promoting holistic healing and personal growth.

The Subconscious Influence on Culture and Society

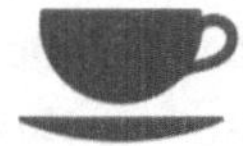

THE SUBCONSCIOUS MIND significantly impacts societal norms, cultural trends, and individual behaviours within a given society. Various mediums, such as advertising, media, and subconscious messaging, actively tap into the subconscious, shaping perceptions, attitudes, and behaviours on a collective scale.

Advertising and Subconscious Messaging

Emotional Appeals and Symbolism

1. Creating Emotional Associations: Advertisements often use imagery and narratives to evoke emotions that create subconscious connections with products or brands.

2. Symbolic Representations: Symbolism in advertisements taps into collective subconscious associations, influencing perceptions and desires.

Subliminal Stimuli and Persuasion

1. Subliminal Messaging: Implicit or hidden messages, though controversial, attempt to influence behaviour or attitudes at a subconscious level.

2. Influencing Consumer Behaviour: Subliminal cues aim to impact decision-making without conscious awareness, subtly shaping consumer choices.

Media Portrayals and Cultural Norms

Reinforcing Stereotypes and Ideals

1. Stereotypical Representations: Media often perpetuates subconscious stereotypes, influencing societal perceptions of gender, race, and social roles.

2. Idealized Images: Portrayals of beauty, success, and lifestyle create subconscious ideals that influence personal aspirations and societal standards.

Cultural Programming and Conditioning

1. Normalization of Behaviours: Repeated exposure to certain behaviours or narratives in media normalizes them, shaping subconscious acceptance or rejection.

2. Shaping Collective Beliefs: Media influences cultural norms by reinforcing or challenging collective beliefs through subconscious messaging.

Social Media and Subconscious Influences

Digital Persuasion Techniques

1. Algorithmic Personalization: Social media platforms employ algorithms that tailor content to individuals, subtly influencing subconscious preferences and behaviours.

2. Peer Influence and Social Norms: Subconscious cues from peers and influencers impact perceptions and decision-making in online environments.

FOMO and Psychological Triggers

1. Fear of Missing Out (FOMO): Subconscious triggers like scarcity tactics or social proof influence behaviours, creating a sense of urgency or conformity.

2. Emotional Responses and Engagement: social media utilizes emotional triggers to capture attention and engagement, influencing subconscious reactions.

Political Messaging and Subconscious Appeals

Framing and Emotional Appeals

1. Framing of Issues: Political messaging employs emotional appeals and framing techniques that resonate with subconscious concerns or aspirations.

2. Influence on Voter Behaviour: Subconscious messaging impacts political choices by appealing to emotions, values, or fears.

Persuasion Strategies

1. Primacy of Emotional Appeals: Political campaigns prioritize emotional connections over rational arguments to influence subconscious decision-making.

2. Subconscious Associations and Bias: Messaging creates subconscious associations with certain candidates or ideologies, influencing voter biases.

Subconscious Resistance and Awareness

Developing Media Literacy

1. Critical Thinking Skills: Developing media literacy helps individuals recognize and decode subconscious messaging techniques used in advertising and media.

2. Awareness of Persuasion Tactics: Understanding subconscious influences empowers individuals to resist manipulation and make informed choices.

Ethical Implications and Regulation

1. Ethical Responsibility: Media and advertisers face ethical dilemmas regarding subconscious manipulation and the impact on societal perceptions and behaviours.

2. Regulatory Measures: Debate surrounds the need for regulations to address subconscious messaging tactics in media and advertising.

The subconscious significantly shapes societal norms, cultural attitudes, and individual behaviours, often influenced by advertising, media, and subconscious messaging. Advertising employs emotional appeals, symbolism, and subliminal cues to influence consumer behaviour. Media portrayals perpetuate stereotypes, shape cultural ideals, and influence social norms through repeated messaging. Social media platforms leverage algorithms and psychological triggers to influence user behaviour and perceptions. Political messaging targets subconscious emotions and values, impacting voter behaviour. Developing media literacy and awareness of subconscious influences empower individuals to discern and resist manipulative tactics. Ethical considerations and debates around regulation arise concerning subconscious messaging's impact on societal perceptions and behaviours. Understanding the subconscious's role in society fosters critical awareness, facilitating informed decision-making and fostering a more conscious and responsible media and advertising landscape.

Ethical Implications of Subconscious Influence

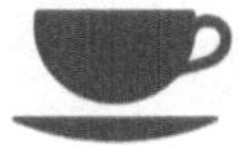

THE UTILIZATION OF subconscious influence in various spheres, including advertising, media, politics, and psychology, raises significant ethical considerations. Understanding the impact of subconscious persuasion prompts discussions on responsibility, transparency, and the ethical boundaries of employing tactics that influence individuals' thoughts, behaviours, and decisions without their explicit awareness.

Informed Consent and Autonomy

Transparency in Messaging

1. Disclosure of Persuasion Tactics: Ethical communication necessitates transparency in revealing subconscious messaging techniques used in advertising, media, and psychological interventions.

2. Respecting Individual Autonomy: Individuals should have the autonomy to make informed decisions, free from manipulative subconscious influences.

Protecting Vulnerable Populations

1. Children and Vulnerable Audiences: Ethical considerations demand safeguarding vulnerable groups from subconscious manipulation due to their heightened susceptibility.

2. Regulating Targeted Marketing: Regulations and ethical guidelines are needed to protect

vulnerable populations from targeted subconscious persuasion tactics.

Consumer Rights and Responsibility

Respecting Consumer Choices

1. Freedom of Choice: Ethical marketing respects consumers' rights by avoiding manipulation and allowing informed decision-making.

2. Balancing Persuasion and Honesty: Adherence to ethical standards requires striking a balance between persuasive messaging and factual honesty.

Avoiding Deceptive Practices

1. Truthfulness in Messaging: Ethical considerations emphasize refraining from deceptive practices that manipulate perceptions or induce false beliefs through subconscious means.

2. Ensuring Ethical Advertising: Adhering to ethical standards prevents exploiting subconscious vulnerabilities for commercial gain.

Psychological Well-being and Harm

Potential for Psychological Harm

1. Unintended Consequences: Subconscious messaging may induce stress, anxiety, or insecurities, raising concerns about psychological well-being.

2. Mitigating Negative Impact: Ethical responsibility involves minimizing potential harm caused by subconscious influences in media or advertising.

Promoting Positive Impact

1. Ethical Persuasion for Social Good: Subconscious messaging can be used ethically to promote positive behaviours, such as health-related changes, without causing harm.

2. Empowerment and Education: Ethical applications of subconscious influence empower individuals through education and positive messaging rather than manipulation.

Professional Responsibility in Psychology

Therapist-Client Relationship

1. Informed Consent in Therapy: Ethical guidelines in psychology mandate informing clients about therapeutic methods involving the subconscious and obtaining consent.

2. Avoiding Coercion or Exploitation: Ethical therapists prioritize client well-being, avoiding coercion or exploitation through subconscious techniques.

Therapeutic Integrity

1. Maintaining Professional Boundaries: Ethical therapists prioritize clients' welfare, refraining from using subconscious persuasion for personal gain or influence.

2. Respecting Client Autonomy: Ethical practitioners respect clients' autonomy and decision-making, avoiding imposing subconscious suggestions without consent.

Regulation and Industry Standards

Ethical Codes and Guidelines

1. Industry Standards: Establishing and adhering to ethical codes and guidelines in advertising, media, and psychology regulates the use of subconscious influence.

2. Oversight and Accountability: Regulatory bodies ensure accountability, monitoring compliance with ethical standards in professional practice and advertising.

Public Awareness and Education

1. Promoting Media Literacy: Ethical considerations emphasize educating the public about subconscious persuasion, fostering critical thinking and resistance to manipulation.

2. Debates on Regulation: Public discourse and debates regarding regulation of subconscious messaging tactics guide ethical policymaking and industry practices.

Utilizing subconscious influence raises ethical questions concerning transparency, autonomy, consumer rights, psychological well-being, and professional responsibility. Ethical considerations necessitate transparency in messaging, protecting vulnerable populations, and respecting consumer autonomy in decision-making. The avoidance of deceptive practices, minimizing psychological harm, and leveraging subconscious persuasion for positive impact align with ethical principles. In psychology, therapists have a responsibility to maintain professional integrity, respect client autonomy, and avoid coercion or exploitation. Regulation and industry standards play a crucial role in ensuring adherence to ethical codes and guidelines. Public awareness and education about subconscious influence foster critical thinking and informed decision-making, empowering individuals to recognize and resist manipulative tactics. Ethical debates and discussions drive policymaking, guiding the responsible use of subconscious persuasion in various fields, promoting ethical practices that prioritize individual autonomy, well-being, and informed consent.

The Subconscious Mind from Spiritual Perspectives

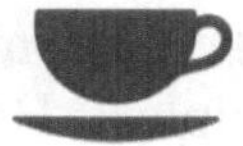

IN SPIRITUAL PHILOSOPHIES and practices worldwide, the subconscious mind holds a significant place, often intertwined with concepts of higher consciousness, spirituality, and the interconnectedness of all beings. Various spiritual traditions interpret the subconscious as a gateway to profound insights, self-realization, and a connection to higher realms or universal consciousness.

Eastern Philosophies and the Subconscious

Yogic and Vedic Views

1. Chitta and Cosmic Consciousness: In yoga and Vedanta, the subconscious, termed "chitta," stores impressions and experiences, with deeper layers connecting to cosmic consciousness or the collective unconscious.

2. Meditation and Self-Realization: Practices like meditation aim to transcend the subconscious mind, leading to self-realization and union with higher states of consciousness.

Buddhism and Awareness

1. Alaya-Vijnana: In Buddhism, the alaya-vijnana, the storehouse consciousness, contains karmic imprints and influences perceptions, fostering mindfulness and awareness to transcend its conditioning.

2. Enlightenment and Liberation: Buddhists seek liberation from the subconscious's grip through mindfulness practices to achieve enlightenment.

Western Esoteric Traditions

Hermeticism and the Unconscious

1. Hermetic Principles: Hermeticism views the subconscious as the repository of hidden knowledge and divine wisdom, suggesting techniques to access and integrate higher truths.

2. Alchemy and Inner Transformation: Alchemical symbolism often refers to the subconscious transformation paralleling spiritual evolution and attainment.

Kabbalistic Perspectives

1. The Kabbalistic Tree of Life: The subconscious, represented in Kabbalah's lower realms, reflects the fragmented aspects of the divine, aiming for integration and unity with higher spiritual spheres.

2. Tikkun HaNefesh: Rectifying the subconscious involves spiritual repair and harmonization of the fragmented soul.

Unity and Oneness

Interconnectedness and Unity Consciousness

1. Collective Unconscious: Spiritually, the collective unconscious represents the interconnectedness of all beings, suggesting that individual subconscious realms are part of a larger, unified consciousness.

2. Universal Wisdom and Insights: Accessing higher levels of the subconscious leads to profound spiritual insights, intuitive wisdom, and a sense of universal interconnectedness.

Connection to Higher Realms and Divinity
Higher Self and Divine Connection

1. Higher Self Realization: Spiritual teachings often emphasize transcending the limitations of the subconscious to connect with the higher self, representing a divine aspect within.

2. Divine Guidance and Intuition: By quieting the subconscious mind, individuals may access spiritual guidance or intuitive insights from higher realms.

Spiritual Practices and Subconscious Exploration
Meditation and Spiritual Growth

1. Contemplative Practices: Meditation and prayer quiet the subconscious chatter, allowing individuals to connect with deeper spiritual realms and achieve inner stillness.

2. Surrender and Letting Go: Spiritual surrender involves relinquishing subconscious attachments and ego identification, facilitating spiritual growth.

Dreamwork and Symbolism

1. Dream Interpretation: In spiritual traditions, dreams carry symbolic messages from the subconscious or higher realms, guiding individuals on their spiritual paths.

2. Symbolic Insights: Understanding dream symbolism offers insights into spiritual growth, facilitating self-awareness and transformation.

Spiritual perspectives on the subconscious highlight its role as a bridge to higher consciousness, divine connection, and spiritual growth. Across diverse traditions, the subconscious is seen as a repository of knowledge, impressions, and karmic imprints, holding the potential for spiritual transformation and self-realization. Practices like meditation, dreamwork, and spiritual surrender aim to transcend the limitations of the subconscious, accessing deeper spiritual truths and interconnectedness with the divine. The exploration and integration of the subconscious within spiritual contexts provide pathways toward inner transformation, unity consciousness, and alignment with higher realms of existence, fostering a deeper understanding of the interconnected nature of all beings and the divine within.

Advances in Subconscious Studies

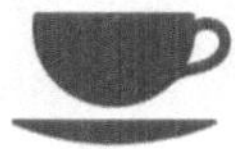

CURRENT RESEARCH AND Future Prospects

In recent years, advancements in neuroscience, psychology, and related fields have led to significant strides in understanding the subconscious mind. Cutting-edge research, innovative technologies, and interdisciplinary approaches are unravelling the complexities of subconscious processes, opening new avenues for exploration and offering insights into human cognition, behaviour, and well-being.

Neuroscientific Insights

Brain Imaging Techniques

1. Functional MRI (fMRI): Advancements in fMRI technology allow researchers to observe brain activity associated with subconscious processes, unveiling neural correlates of subconscious thoughts, emotions, and decision-making.

2. EEG and Neurofeedback: Electroencephalography (EEG) combined with neurofeedback techniques offers real-time monitoring and regulation of subconscious brain activity, aiding in therapeutic interventions.

Subconscious Processing

1. Implicit Learning: Studying implicit learning processes sheds light on how the subconscious acquires and applies information without conscious awareness, influencing behaviour and decision-making.

2. Subliminal Perception: Research explores the thresholds and mechanisms of subliminal perception, uncovering how minimal stimuli impact subconscious processing.

Behavioural Psychology and Subconscious Influences

Automatic Behaviours and Habits

1. Habit Formation: Understanding subconscious habit formation aids in behaviour modification and interventions targeting automatic responses linked to the subconscious.

2. Behavioural Priming: Investigating behavioural priming effects reveals how subtle cues influence subconscious decision-making and actions.

Unconscious Bias and Decision-Making

1. Implicit Bias Studies: Research on unconscious biases and their impact on decision-making offers insights into mitigating biases and fostering inclusivity.

2. Ethical Implications: Exploring ethical considerations of subconscious biases guides interventions to minimize unintended discriminatory effects.

Artificial Intelligence and Machine Learning

AI-Based Subconscious Analysis

1. Pattern Recognition: Machine learning algorithms analyse patterns in subconscious responses, predicting behaviours or preferences based on subtle cues.

2. Personalized Recommendations: AI-driven systems use subconscious data to offer personalized recommendations in various fields, including marketing and healthcare.

Cognitive Computing

1. Natural Language Processing: Cognitive computing applications interpret and respond to language cues, incorporating subconscious linguistic nuances in interactions.

2. Emotionally Intelligent Systems: AI systems simulate emotional understanding, recognizing and responding to subtle subconscious emotional cues.

Psychodynamic and Therapeutic Innovations

Advanced Therapeutic Techniques

1. Neuro-Psychotherapy: Integrating neuroscientific findings into psychotherapy improves interventions, targeting subconscious processes for therapeutic benefits.

2. Virtual Reality Therapy: VR-based interventions explore subconscious responses to immersive experiences, aiding in exposure therapy and trauma treatment.

Subconscious Reprogramming

1. Precision Mental Health: Tailored interventions based on individual subconscious traits or neural patterns optimize reprogramming strategies for personalized outcomes.

2. Innovative Hypnotherapy: Advancements in hypnosis techniques leverage neuroscience to enhance subconscious access and therapeutic outcomes.

Future Prospects and Ethical Considerations

Brain-Computer Interfaces

1. Enhanced Communication: Developing BCIs for subconscious communication might facilitate direct interaction, benefiting individuals with limited verbal or conscious abilities.

2. Ethical Challenges: Addressing ethical dilemmas surrounding privacy, consent, and potential misuse of subconscious data remains crucial in BCI development.

Ethical AI and Subconscious Manipulation

1. Guardrails in AI Development: Ethical guidelines are imperative to prevent AI systems from exploiting subconscious vulnerabilities for manipulation or harm.

2. Regulation and Transparency: Advocating for regulations ensuring transparency and accountability in AI applications involving subconscious data protects users from manipulation.

Interdisciplinary Collaboration and Knowledge Integration

Convergence of Fields

1. Neuro-ethics and Subconscious Studies: Collaboration between neuro-ethicists and subconscious researchers navigates ethical complexities in subconscious exploration and applications.

2. Holistic Integration: Interdisciplinary approaches merging neuroscience, psychology, ethics, and technology foster comprehensive understanding and responsible application of subconscious studies.

Advances in subconscious studies driven by neuroscience, psychology, artificial intelligence, and therapeutic innovations have unveiled the intricacies of subconscious processes. Cutting-edge technologies, such as brain imaging, AI-driven analyses, and therapeutic interventions, offer insights into subconscious mechanisms, influencing behaviour, decision-making, and well-being. Future prospects revolve around brain-computer interfaces, ethical AI development, and interdisciplinary collaborations, aiming to navigate ethical dilemmas, enhance therapeutic interventions, and explore the frontiers of subconscious exploration responsibly. The convergence of fields and holistic integration of knowledge promise to shape the future of subconscious studies, fostering a deeper understanding of human cognition, behaviour, and the ethical implications of subconscious research and applications.

Reflection on the Subconscious Mind

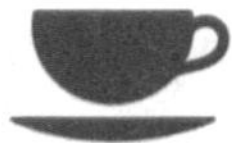

THE EXPLORATION OF the subconscious mind across the preceding chapters has illuminated its multifaceted nature, unveiling its profound impact on human cognition, behaviour, and the intricate interplay between conscious and subconscious processes. Reflecting on key insights, implications, and the future trajectory of subconscious studies offers a comprehensive understanding of its significance and potential applications.

Understanding the Subconscious

Nature and Mechanisms

1. Depth and Complexity: The subconscious operates beyond conscious awareness, storing memories, emotions, and automatic processes shaping our thoughts and behaviours.

2. Influence on Behaviour: It exerts a pervasive influence, guiding decision-making, habits, emotions, and responses to stimuli without direct conscious involvement.

Interconnectedness with Consciousness

1. Duality of Consciousness: The interplay between conscious and subconscious processes forms a dynamic relationship, influencing perceptions and shaping experiences.

2. Integration and Symbiosis: Understanding and integrating subconscious elements into conscious

awareness fosters holistic self-awareness and personal growth.

Significance and Implications

Practical Applications

1. Therapeutic Interventions: Subconscious-focused therapies and techniques aid in addressing deep-seated issues, reprogramming beliefs, and fostering psychological well-being.

2. Advertising and Influence: Insights into subconscious mechanisms inform marketing strategies, media communications, and political messaging, influencing societal perceptions and behaviours.

Ethical Considerations

1. Responsibility and Transparency: Ethical implications of subconscious influence call for transparency, respecting autonomy, and safeguarding vulnerable populations from manipulation.

2. Regulation and Oversight: Establishing ethical guidelines and regulations ensures the responsible use of subconscious techniques in various fields.

Future Trajectory and Possibilities

Advancements and Research

1. Neuroscientific Innovations: Advancements in brain imaging, artificial intelligence, and cognitive research offer deeper insights into subconscious processes and their neural correlates.

2. Integration of Disciplines: Interdisciplinary collaboration fosters a comprehensive understanding of the subconscious, exploring innovative applications and ethical frameworks.

Holistic Integration and Well-being

1.   Psychological   Well-being: Harnessing subconscious processes promotes mental health, self-awareness, and personal growth through therapeutic interventions and self-reflection.

2. Spiritual and Holistic Perspectives: Bridging spiritual philosophies with subconscious studies offers avenues for self-realization, higher consciousness, and interconnectedness.

The journey through the exploration of the subconscious mind has unveiled its profound influence on human cognition, behaviour, and societal dynamics. The complexity of subconscious mechanisms, their interconnectedness with consciousness, and their practical applications across various fields underscore the significance of understanding and responsibly harnessing its power.

Reflection on the ethical implications emphasizes the need for transparency, ethical guidelines, and regulatory measures to safeguard against potential manipulation and protect individual autonomy. The convergence of neuroscience, psychology, technology, and ethical considerations promises a future marked by innovative research, interdisciplinary collaboration, and holistic applications beneficial for individual well-being and societal progress.

The subconscious mind stands as a gateway to self-discovery, personal growth, and a deeper understanding of human nature. Its exploration, ethical application, and integration into diverse spheres of life hold immense potential for shaping a future that honours individual autonomy, promotes well-being, and fosters a deeper connection between the conscious self and the vast depths of the subconscious realm. As we continue to unravel its mysteries, the subconscious mind remains an intriguing frontier, offering boundless possibilities for exploration, understanding, and transformation.

The claustrum is a thin, irregular sheet of neurons deep within the brain. Francis Crick, along with his colleague Christof Koch, proposed that the claustrum might play a crucial role in integrating information across different brain regions, contributing to consciousness. This theory emerged from Crick's and Koch's investigations into the neural correlates of consciousness.

The claustrum's exact function is still not fully understood, but it is believed to have connections to many regions of the cerebral cortex. It appears to act as a hub, orchestrating communication between various brain regions.

- Brief overview of Francis Crick's work and his contributions to neuroscience.

- Introduction to the claustrum: its anatomical location, structure, and historical understanding.

- Establish the significance of the claustrum in the context of consciousness and brain function.

Anatomy and Connectivity of the Claustrum

- Detailed description of the claustrum's anatomical features.

- Explanation of its connectivity with other brain regions, including the cortex and subcortical structures.

- Discuss how its connectivity patterns suggest a role in integrating information from various brain areas.

Francis Crick's Hypothesis on the Claustrum and Consciousness

- Explanation of Crick's proposal regarding the claustrum's role in consciousness.

- Elaborate on Crick and Koch's attention to the claustrum's connectivity and how it could integrate information.

- Discuss how their theory aimed to bridge the gap between neural activity and subjective experience.

Supporting Evidence and Research

- Review studies and experiments that support Crick's hypothesis.

- Explore neuroimaging or neurophysiological evidence suggesting the involvement of the claustrum in coordinating brain activity.

Critiques and Alternative Views

- Discuss criticisms or challenges to Crick's hypothesis.

- Present alternative theories about the claustrum's function and its relation to consciousness.

- Address limitations in research methodologies or conflicting findings in the field.

Recent Advances and Future Directions

- Review recent studies or technological advancements that shed light on the claustrum's function.

- Discuss the potential future directions in claustrum research and methodologies to investigate its role in consciousness.

- Summarize key points regarding the claustrum's function and its relation to consciousness.

- Emphasize the ongoing debate and the importance of further research in understanding the claustrum's role in brain function and consciousness.

Remember, this is an outline, and a comprehensive idea on the claustrum and consciousness would require an in-depth review of scientific literature, research findings, and critical analysis of the proposed theories.

Don't miss out!

Click the button below and you can sign up to receive emails whenever Jagdish Krishanlal Arora publishes a new book. There's no charge and no obligation.

Did you love *Subconcious Programming*? Then you should read *Motivation* by Jagdish Krishanlal Arora et al.!

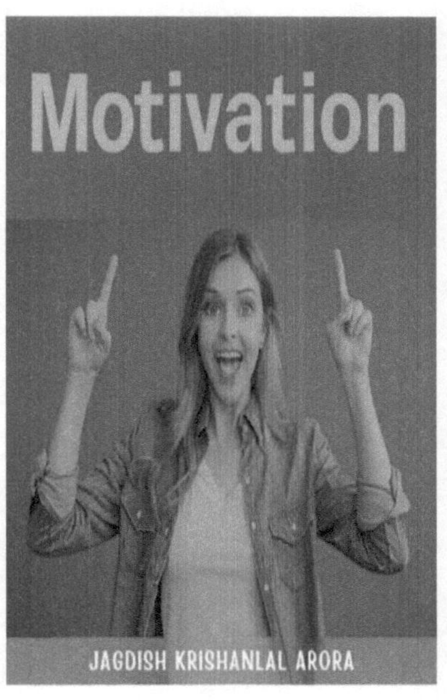

Motivation refers to the psychological processes that drive and direct our behavior towards achieving certain goals or fulfilling specific needs. It is the force that energizes, sustains, and guides our actions, thoughts, and emotions. Motivation can arise from various sources, including internal factors like personal values, interests, and aspirations, as well as external factors like rewards, recognition, and social pressure. It plays a crucial role in influencing our decisions, shaping our attitudes, and determining the level of effort we invest in tasks. Different theories of motivation, such as Maslow's hierarchy of needs, expectancy theory, and self-determination theory, provide insights into understanding the complexities of human motivation and how it impacts behavior.

Also by Jagdish Krishanlal Arora

<u>Basic Inorganic and Organic Chemistry</u>
<u>Book of Jokes</u>
<u>Car Insurance and Claims</u>
<u>Digital Electronics, Computer Architecture and Microprocessor Design Principles</u>
<u>Guided Meditation and Yoga</u>
<u>The Bible and Jesus Christ</u>
<u>Unity Quest</u>
<u>From Oasis to Global Stage: The Evolution of Arab Civilization</u>
<u>Secrets of Mount Kailash, Bermuda Triangle and the Lost City of Atlantis</u>
<u>Visitors from Outer Space</u>
<u>Motivation</u>
<u>The Aliens and God Theory</u>
<u>The Lunar Voyager</u>
<u>Queen Elizabeth II and the British Monarchy</u>
<u>The Kremlin Conspiracy</u>
<u>Vegetable Gardening, Salads and Recipes</u>
<u>How to End The War in Ukraine</u>
<u>The Old and New World Order</u>
<u>Travelling to Mars in the Cosmic Odyssey 2050</u>
<u>Romance Pays Off</u>
<u>How the Universe Works</u>
<u>Mental Health and Well Being</u>
<u>Ancient History of Mars</u>
<u>The Nexus</u>
<u>Basic and Advanced Physics</u>

Administrative Law
Calculus
The Ramayana
A Watery Mystery
Romantic Conflicts
Thieves of Palestine
Love in Chicago
WordPress Design and Development
Travellers Guide to Mount Kailash
Become a Better Writer With Creative Writing
Emerging Trends in Carbon Emission Reduction
India Independence Through Non Violence
Copyright, Patents, Trademarks and Trade Secret Laws
Decoding CHATGPT and Artificial Intelligence
The Untold Story of Diana and Prince Charles
Time Travel
How to Lose Weight Quickly
Subconcious Programming